MAKE KEFIR WITH EASE

AN ILLUSTRATIVE AND DESCRIPTIVE GUIDE WITH AMAZING PICTURES ON HOW TO BREW KEFIR FOR NATURAL HEALING

HUMPHREY JACK

Table of Contents

CHAPTER ONE

INTRODUCTION

Water kefir is a sort of refreshment drink that is supported for the two its bubbly flavor and general medical advantages. It started in the late 1800s. It is known for its amazing punch of probiotics. It is an exceptionally delicious beverage that has been appeared to amp up invulnerability; improve wellbeing and moderate disease cell development. It is so energizing to realize that water kefir can be made at home in only scarcely any means and with hardly any fixings.

What Is Water Kefir?

Water kefir is a sort of refreshment delivered from kefir grains. It is matured and carbonated refreshment. Water kefir is otherwise called japanese water gems, tibicos, California honey bees and a few different names.

Dissimilar to different sorts of kefir produced using the milk of goat, dairy animals or sheep, water kefir is created by a blend of water kefir grains and sugar water. Water kefir grains comprise of a sort of grain-like culture of yeast and microscopic organisms.

The blend is gotten by aging for around 24 to 48 hours. This blend along these lines creates a probiotic drink that is wealthy in gainful microscopic organisms.

Water kefir is delectable and simple to make. It likewise contains a few medical advantages that can be a great expansion to a balanced nutritious dinner.

CHAPTER TWO

ADVANTAGE OF WATER KEFIR

1.   Rich in Beneficial Bacteria

A noteworthy advantage of water kefir is the way that it is wealthy in probiotic content. Probiotic is a sort of useful microbes generally found in the gut and it assumes a basic job in pretty much every part of wellbeing. It assists with forestalling malignancy and furthermore helps resistance. The facts confirm that yogurt is the famous wellspring of probiotics, in any case, the cutting edge kefir is really viewed as a superior wellspring of probiotics. This is on the grounds that it gives a differing scope of yeast and microscopic organisms. Indeed, even some exploration shows that kefir grains contain in excess of 50 diverse yeast and bacterial strains. The following are the absolute most basic groups of helpful microorganisms found in kefir, they are

- Lactobacillus

- Lactococcus

- Streptococcus

- Leuconostoc

- Bifidobacterium

- Thermophilus

- Bulgaricus

- Helveticus

2.   May Help Fight Cancer Cells

The exploration anyway is restricted to test-tube examines. This exploration proposes that water kefir can assist with diminishing the development of particular sorts of malignancy. One of the examination found that extricates from kefir is powerful at obstructing the development of bosom malignancy cells. Then, some different investigations did demonstrate that kefir is really valuable against blood malignancy and colon. This is seen as obvious on the grounds that it is extremely wealthy in probiotics. It additionally assists with boosting resistant capacities that help to help malignancy anticipation. Be that as it may, there might be requirement for more research to assess this evidence.

3.   Could Boost Immune Function

Because of the high convergence of useful microbes, adding water kefir to your eating regimen every day can assist with boosting your resistant framework extraordinarily. Studies and research completed on people demonstrated that specific strains of probiotics could truly help in diminishing your danger of respiratory contaminations, intestinal diseases and furthermore the anticipation of urinary tract diseases in ladies. Research and studies completed in creatures indicated that kefir can likewise assist with stifling fiery reactions that are activated by issues, for example, asthma.

Another little six-week study did in 18 individuals indicated that expending kefir every day had the option to help in controlling aggravation and improve levels of invulnerable cells in the body.

4.   Dairy-Free and Vegan

The conventional method of making kefir is by utilizing dairy animals or goat milk joined with kefir grains. This delivers a thick, probiotic rich refreshment. Be that as it may, since the creation of water kefir utilizing sugar water, it is a generally excellent preferred position for the individuals who decide to stay away from dairy, possibly because of individual reasons, medical problems or dietary limitations. It is simply ideal for probiotic and boosting your gut wellbeing for those following a dairy free or veggie lover diet so as limit your utilization of creature items.

5. May Cause Side Effects in Some People

Water kefir can be securely delighted in by a few people without any dangers of any unfavorable impacts. In any case, some normal reactions related with it are stomach related problems, for example, swelling, queasiness, issues and blockage. These symptoms vanish when utilization proceeds. Individuals with powerless safe framework, for example, AID patients should check with their PCP before utilizing water kefir.

6. Easy to make and appreciate at Home

Water kefir is a seasoned drink that is anything but difficult to make. It has a few medical advantages that are useful for your body. Despite the fact that the taste may change because of a few factors yet the wonderful thing about it is that it tastes marginally sweet with somewhat of a level delayed flavor impression.

CHAPTER THREE

EASY STEPS TO MAKE WATER KEFIR AT HOME

Consolidate 1/2 cup (118 ml) of high temp water along with 1/4 cup (50 grams) of sugar in a bowl or container.

• Swirl the blend together to break down.

• Add around 3 cups (710 ml) of room temperature water to the bowl or container

• Add your water kefir grains.

• Cover and spot the bowl or container in a warm zone with a temperature of around 68 to 85°F (20 to 30°C) and permit to age for around 24 to 48 hours.

•   Next is to isolate the water kefir grains from the blend

•   Add another bunch of sugar water (the finished item is prepared for your utilization and satisfaction).

•   You can decide to drink the water kefir all things considered or include flavors, for example, organic product juice, mint leaves, vanilla concentrate or solidified natural products

WHAT ARE WATER KEFIR GRAINS?

A few people know about milk kefir grains, however not water kefir grains. It is deserving of note that the two items are produced using "grains". Be that as it may, these grains are not genuine grains like wheat or rye. These grains are groups of yeast and microorganisms and living in a harmonious relationship that are held together by a polysaccharide (dextran) that is created by Lactobacillus higarii. The groups of microorganisms, yeast, and polysaccharide take after little precious stones, or "grains" of jam. The yeast and microscopic organisms present in the grains utilizes sugar to create carbon dioxide, lactic corrosive and ethanol (limited quantity).

NAMES FOR WATER KEFIR GRAINS

Water kefir grains are called by an assortment of names. Most normally called are Japanese water gems, tibicos, and California honey bees. They are likewise alluded to as ocean rice, Australian Bees, water pearls, African Bees, Ginger Bees, Ginger

Beer Plant to specify however a couple. Water kefir has various names in different nations. They are called piltz in Germany and are called Kefir di Frutta in Italy and are called Graines Vivantes in Mexico. The microscopic organisms and yeasts in water kefir grains are dynamic. It is imperative to take note of that there are numerous varieties of the specific culture that creates the bubbly water kefir refreshment drink.

THE ORIGIN OF WATER KEFIR

Where water kefir grains started from isn't totally clear. In any case, theories have it that it began from Mexico. A few research have it that the tibicos culture that is created on the stack of the Opuntia desert flora as hard granules that can be reconstituted in a sugar-water arrangement as proliferating tibicos. There is anyway documentation from the late 1800s in Mexico of water kefir grains utilized as a matured beverage that was produced using an improved juice of the thorny pear desert plant. A few stories anyway puts their cause, or their uses in Tibet, the Caucasus Mountains, the southern promontory of the Ukraine. To pinpoint a precise spot where water kefir started from is troublesome on the grounds that water kefir societies are discovered everywhere throughout the world and no two societies are actually same. There was no written history, this has made it hard to put an inception date. Research demonstrated that these grains have been utilized for a long time.

Names for water kefir

- Tibicos   (Tibi)
- Búlgaros
- Bees
- Japanese Water Crystals
- Japanese Beer seeds
- Graines Vivantes (French)
- Wasserkefir
- Sugar Kefir Grains
- Piltz, (German)
- Kefir di Frutta (Italian)
- Kefirs/Keefir/Kephir
- Aqua Gems
- Sea   Rice
- Sugary   Fungus

- Kefir d'acqua/water

- Kefir d'uva (grape juice is utilized)

- Bébées

- African bees

- California Bees

- Australian bees

- Vinegar bees

- Ginger bees

- Ale nuts

- Balm of Gilead

- Beer seeds

- Beer plant

CHAPTER FOUR

STEP BY STEP INSTRUCTIONS TO USE WATER KEFIR GRAINS

The technique for utilizing water kefir grains are essentially the equivalent all through the world regardless of the different names given to water kefir grains. They are fundamentally utilized by adding them to a sugar water and afterward permit the way of life on the counter to mature for a day or two to get a bubbly, aged beverage.

THE TWO TYPES OF KEFIR

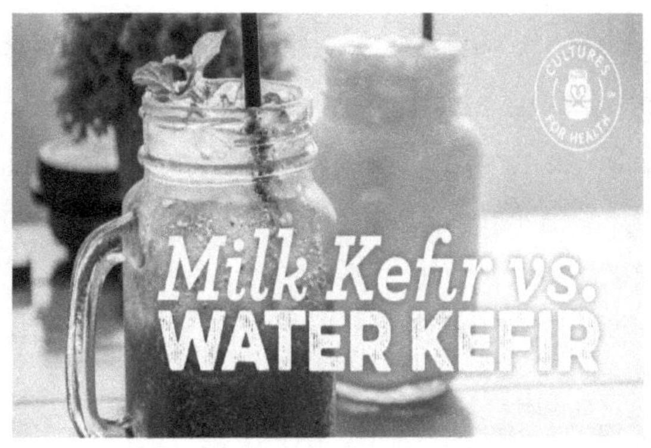

MILK KEFIR AND WATER KEFIR

There are fundamentally two distinct sorts of kefir.

•   Milk kefir: It is a probiotic refreshment that is notable and can be found in numerous markets.

•   Water kefir: it is additionally a probiotic-rich drink. The thing that matters is that water kefir is sans dairy and a lighter drink and it takes into account enhancing in a few different ways.

N.B. Both sort of kefir have their own interesting attributes however they are made marginally in an unexpected way. On the off chance that you want to add probiotics to your day by day normal, at that point keep an eye out for which of these matured refreshments is best for you.

DISTINCTION BETWEEN MILK KEFIR AND WATER KEFIR

Milk Kefir

Milk kefir is delivered from dairy animals milk, goat milk, or coconut milk. You can likewise make it with other non-dairy milks. This may anyway create a conflicting outcome.

Water Kefir

Water kefir then again is made with sugar water, natural product juice and kefir grains. Water kefir may likewise require a starter culture. You may choose to utilize a Kefir Starter Culture or Water Kefir Grains; everything relies upon how frequently you need to make water kefir.

WHAT KEFIR CONTAINS

Milk Kefir Grains comprise of a customary reusable starter culture that is utilized to make a probiotic-rich drink with live dynamic yeast and microscopic organisms.

Water Kefir Grains then again are likewise customary reusable starter cultures that are utilized to make dairy free refined refreshment with live dynamic microorganisms and yeast.

HOW DOES KEFIR TASTE?

Milk Kefir

Milk kefir has a possess a flavor like that of refined milk. The flavor of each clump created be that as it may, relies upon the pace of aging. An all around aged kefir can have an exceptionally solid harsh taste and can be somewhat carbonated. While a shorter maturation can give a progressively mellow flavor.

Water Kefir

Water kefir then again has a sweet however somewhat matured flavor. A few people inclines toward seasoned water kefir.

HOW TO FLAVOR KEFIR

MILK KEFIR

Milk Kefir can be handily seasoned by mixing it in a new or solidified organic product or flavor concentrates, for example, vanilla, nectar, maple syrup, stevia and so on. A few people lean toward aging their milk kefir a subsequent time to upgrade flavor.

WATER KEFIR

Water Kefir then again can be enhanced utilizing new or dried natural product, flavor concentrates, for example, vanilla, herbs or organic product juice.

DIFFERENT USES OF KEFIR

Milk Kefir grains can be utilized

- To vaccinate cream to make kefir cream or refined margarine.

- Milk kefir grains can likewise be utilized as a starter culture for aging vegetables.

- Extra milk kefir can likewise be utilized to splash flour before heating or sourdough.

Water Kefir can be utilized

- It can be added to non-dairy milk to make a non-dairy kefir.

- Extra water kefir grains can likewise be utilized as starter culture for aging vegetables.

- Extra water kefir can likewise be utilized as a boosting specialist for making without gluten sourdough starter.

CHAPTER FIVE

BREWING PROPER WATER KEFIR

Kefir is a sort of matured beverage that is created from kefir "grains". Kefir grain is a yeast/bacterial maturation starter. It is set up by combining water, sugar blend and kefir grains and permitting it to mature.

Kefir grains comprise of a mix of lactic corrosive yeast and microorganisms in a protein grid just as lipids and sugars.

Stage 1: Gather materials required

The following are a portion of the things that would be expected to make Kefir

1.   Get kefir grains from wellbeing food store

2.   Glass container - around 1 1litre container for 4 tbsp Kefir grains

3.   Bowl (non-metal) to keep grains

4.   Sieve or plastic sifter

5.   Sugar

6.   Dried natural products to take care of grains so they develop

7.   Paper towels or napkins

8.   Rubber groups

9.   Clean spring water without chlorine

10.   Sealable containers to store completed drink

Stage 2: The Sugar Part

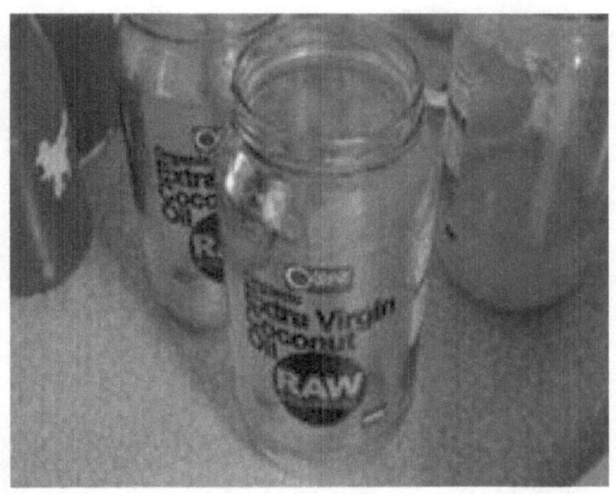

•   Measure out your grains. This will decide how much sugar that will be required.

•   The proportion is 1 tbsp of grains, 1 tbsp of sugar; this will approach 1 Cup of Spring water.

•   Get a huge container that can contain it for (one (1) liter for example 25 gallon/1000ml container with 4 tbsp grains you will require 4 tbsp of sugar).

•   Place this into the base of the container and break down in a limited quantity of warm water.

Stage 3: Add spring Water

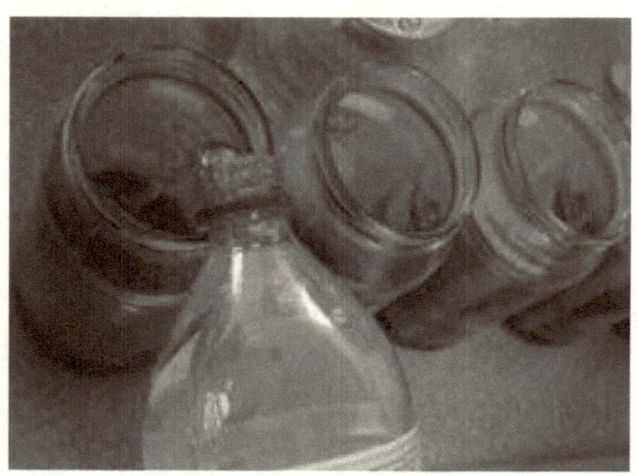

•   Add the spring water; include 1 cup of water

- Pour water into the sugar/water blend

- Stir a little to stir up

Stage 4: Grains

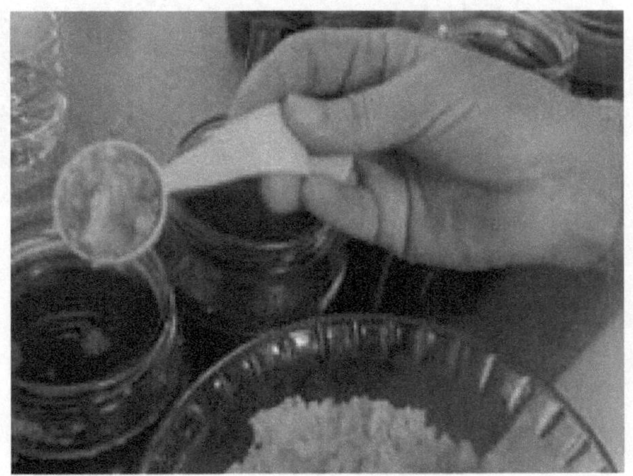

- Add the grains (for 1 liter, include 4 tbsp of grains).

- Pour into the container and permit it to sit or settle.

Stage 5: Brew Time

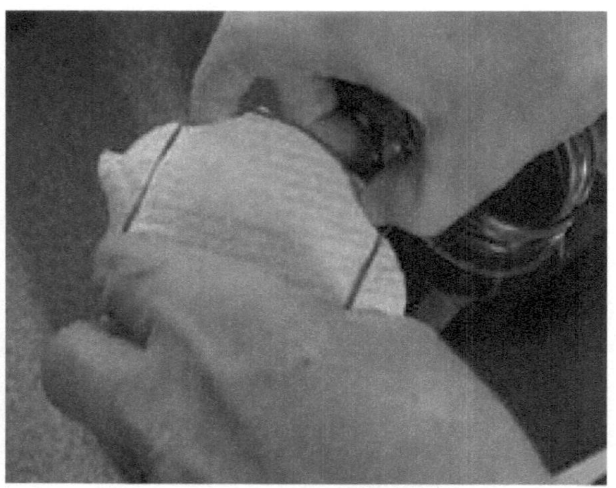

• Next is to cover the containers and permit to sit.

• Cut a paper towel in quarters to get 4 squares (you can on the other hand use muslin).

• Put the towel square over the highest point of the container and secure with an elastic band.

- Next is to set the container aside and permit to blend (permit to mix for 24-48 hours).

In the event that you are new to making water kefir, you may not know precisely what taste you are searching for, yet as you proceed in the creation of water kefir, you will become more acquainted with when to strain the kefir.

Stage 6: Straining Time

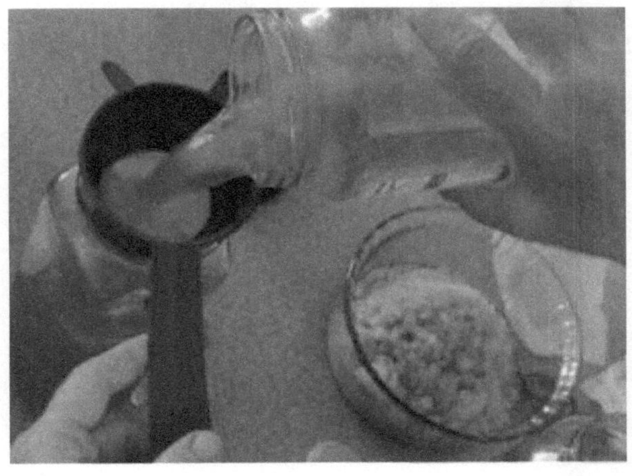

•	At the stage, you can reveal your Kefir and strain it into another container.

•	Ensure your container can hermetically sealed for the second phase of aging.

•	Strain out the grains and set them aside into a non metal bowl to hang tight for the following mix.

•	You can decide to enhance the Kefir at this stage on the off chance that you wish.

•	The second mature can last as long as 24 hours after which your kefir is prepared for drinking.

•	Next is packaging and enhancing of kefir you

N.B. you can re-utilize the grains quickly and start another mix procedure. You can decide to flush or wash the container however this may not be essential without fail. Flush or change jostles when you notice overabundance develop on the grounds that such develop can cause your kefir to age too rapidly and this can make your kefir excessively yeasty and not delicious.

CHAPTER SIX

MEDICAL ADVANTAGES OF DRINKING WATER KEFIR

1. Assists with initiating the Digestive System: Water kefir is extremely helpful for controlling the stomach's acridity and in the enactment of the stomach related framework.

2. Assists with limiting Food Intolerance

Water kefir has an exceptionally positive task to carry out in limiting food narrow mindedness. Nourishments that think that its hard to process don't course in the blood rather they corrupt in the digestive organs. This assists with assuming an immunological job most particularly in adjusting of microbes.

3. Aides Strengthens the Immune System

Water kefir has a positive task to carry out on our insusceptible framework. Water kefir contains a lactic age that have antibacterial impacts and this can assist with offering our body with assurance against illnesses and disease. The probiotic microbes present in water kefir can assist with controlling the inordinate development of pathogens just as the deterioration of microscopic organisms in the digestive system. Water kefir can go about as a characteristic disinfectant and can likewise assist with boosting digestion and cell breath.

4. Water kefir contains Vitamins

Water kefir is a rich wellspring of nutrients. It is plentiful in Vitamin C and nutrient B (B1 and B6). Additionally, natural products added to water kefir contain Vitamin C and other significant supplements.

The Vitamin B1

• Carry out cardiovascular capacities

• Improves cerebrum capacities

• Protects the nerves

• Assist in helping processing

• Protects the mucous layer

• Prevents the advancement of sickliness

- Helps in the amalgamation of glucose.

The Vitamin B6

- Helps to help the resistant framework

- Helps to help cerebrum capacities

- Helps to control issues that are conduct

- Helps to improve our mind-set

- Helps to treat hypertension

- Helps to forestall cardiovascular disorders

- Helps to upgrade digestion

- Helps to help enzymatic framework

Nutrient C

- Helps in the decrease of asthma

- Helps to forestall waterfalls

- Helps to bring down degrees of glycosylated hemoglobin,

- Helps to secure against oxidation of proteins

- Helps to diminish the symptoms of malignant growth chemotherapy

- Helps to help a solid safe framework

5. Decreases Allergic Reactions

The nearness of probiotics in water kefir can assist with forestalling sensitivities just as battling of infections and microscopic organisms. Sensitivities are typically brought about by narrow mindedness to some sort of food eaten. These hypersensitive side effects may shift starting with one individual then onto the next. Water kefir is extremely helpful for diminishing unfavorably susceptible responses.

6. Water Kefir likewise assists with boosting vitality

Water kefir contains a few basic supplements that help to support the vitality level of the body. Including coconut juice to water kefir can help in boosting your vitality levels since coconut juice contains potassium which is valuable in the reinforcing of the muscles.

7. Water kefir as an Anti-Inflammatory specialist

Aggravation happens because of wounds. Irritations essentially are a characteristic method of body reaction to harm. In the event that a physical issue happens in the body or the body gets harmed, the body utilizes aggravations to protect itself from the impact of microorganisms and infection. To do this successfully, the body requires an extra measure of supplements that will help mending process. At the point when water kefir is taken into the body, the minerals and valuable microorganisms present in the water kefir assists with feeding the body. Subsequently, water kefir is a solid calming operator. Water kefir likewise help to mend certain ailments, for example, queasiness, looseness of the bowels and acid reflux.

8. Battles Against Cancer

Drinking water kefir can help a lot in battling against malignant growth. Research and studies have demonstrated that taking water kefir drink normally can help in the anticipation ovarian and bosom disease.

9. Water Kefir Act as an Anti-parasitic and Antibiotic Agent

Drinking water kefir is an exceptionally solid method of ensuring your body. Water kefir is an extremely rich wellspring of probiotic and this makes it a functioning enemy of contagious and anti-toxin specialist. It likewise contains helpful microscopic organisms that empowers it battle against growths and different illnesses

10. Forestalls Diabetes

Since water kefir is a rich wellspring of probiotic, it can help in decreasing the sugar level in the body. This makes it valuable for individuals with diabetes as it assists with forestalling the transition of blood glucose.

11. Treatment of Asthma

Water kefir drink has a constructive outcome in the treatment of asthma because of the nearness of mitigating supplements.

12. Building Bone Density

Water kefir is a rich wellspring of calcium, magnesium which are essential in building of bone density.

THE END